Weight Loss Made Fast and Simple

The 5 Step Guide to Fitness

By Yannick E. Simmons

Table of Contents

Introduction

You wake up in the morning, it is there. You look yourself in the mirror, it is there. You go out, interact with people, it is there. You come home in the evening, it is still there. That feeling that there is something wrong with the way you look. That constant insecurity that follows you everywhere you go, in everything you do. The fear of judgment from people around you. The lack of confidence to approach these people. All these things have been making your life harder than it should be, and the very fact that you are reading this shows that you are yearning for a change. That you are not satisfied with the body you currently have, and that you would like to get in better shape. For yourself, your spouse, your friends, or simply for the whole world to see you differently. So you can feel more confident about the way you look and the way you are perceived by others. Or, maybe you are very comfortable with the way you look but would just like to get in shape for health purposes. In any case, if you feel like some of what I just said applies to you, then you are in luck because it is all about to change. For good. I have come up with a plan for guaranteed weight loss and am about to share it with you. By following the guidelines in this book and applying all the recommended adjustments to your day to day routine, I guarantee you will quickly and naturally find your way to the fit and sexy body you have always dreamed of.

What to Expect from This book?

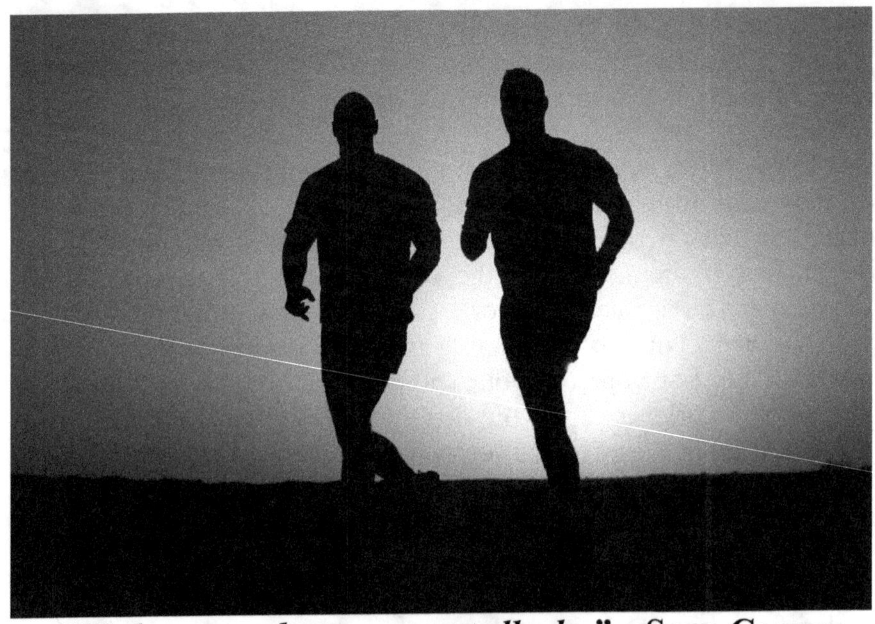

"We become what we repeatedly do." – Sean Covey

Before we go any further, I want to make sure we are all on the same page in terms of what you will get out of this book. This is not your typical, lose x number of pounds in x number of days type of book. It is not filled with facts and details about your metabolism, digestion process, and other scientific weight loss concepts. This is a step by step guide to weight loss for men and women of all ages. It contains a list of rules and lifestyle adjustments you need to implement in order to improve your daily routine, and shape your body to your satisfaction. In time, these adjustments will become habits, and you will lose weight simply by living your life. All the guidelines you will find here come directly from my personal experience losing weight, which is unlike anything I have ever come across on the internet. If you are wondering what is so special about my weight loss plan, the answer is quite simple. It works. Guaranteed. For the past three years, I have been working as a fitness coach, helping men and women lose significant amounts of weight. I have done so using the exact same methods described in this book, and the results have been phenomenal so far. Furthermore, most of these people were able to master this new weight loss routine within just weeks. Keep in mind that there is no set duration or time limit to this plan I have for you. Like I said, it is a routine. You are free to follow it for as long as you desire, depending on what your weight loss goals are. All you have to do is be honest with yourself and thoroughly apply all the necessary adjustments.

Who am I? My Journey from Fat to Fit

My name is Yannick Simmons, and I am a 175 pounds 6 feet tall healthy man. Five years ago, I never would have dreamed of saying that about myself. The year was 2011, one of the most important years of my life. The year I changed and became the person I am today. The year I lost 60 pounds in just 8 months. Yes, 60 pounds! Indeed, I used to weigh 235 pounds. I was clearly overweight and had been for most of my life. I was very aware of the fact that I was different, and thus extremely self-conscious. I actually believe that being different is a blessing. Our differences make us unique and our uniqueness enriches the world, making it an interesting place to be. But some of these differences can be very detrimental, especially when they impact factors of our day to day happiness. Did being overweight make me unhappy? Definitely. And as a result of that unhappiness, I always resorted to unhealthy sources of temporary pleasure such as party size bags of Cheetos, which, inevitably, led to me putting on more weight, and feeling more depressed. In other words, I was caught in the middle of a cheesy crunchy vicious cycle with no plans for escape. And I kept asking myself. Why me? Why am I so fat? Why can't I lose weight? With all the fit and skinny looking dudes out there, how come I am one of the overweight ones?

And so I woke up one day and decided it was time for a change. I did what most people in this situation do. I went on google and looked up "How to lose weight fast". Like I said before, the internet is full of facts and articles about weight loss, diets, metabolism and all that. So I spent hours researching ways to lose weight and tried them for a short while. I tried dieting for a few weeks, but could never stick to one meal plan. I tried exercising but could never do it consistently. In other words, I did not have the patience nor the discipline to lose weight. And no matter how many times I tried, I would always go back to eating chicken wings and fries while watching an episode of The Walking Dead at 2 in the morning.

And then one day something incredible happened. After having had yet another disgusting dinner, I borrowed my roommate's scale just so I could measure how fat and gross I felt. A few seconds after stepping on it, I was shocked. I weighed 235 pounds! Keep in mind that I am only 6 feet tall. Being able to put a number on my excessive weight was a serious reality check. I knew I was big but had no idea how big. I have to say it was a little depressing. However, I did something completely unexpected that night. I put on my old and unused running shoes and went to the gym for a run. As I was completely out of shape, I did not run much and spent most of my time at the gym walking around the jogging track. Then I went home, showered, and went to sleep. Depressed and disappointed. I woke up the next morning with the same feeling, and the first thing I did was step on my roommate's scale again. And again, I was shocked. Only this time, in an awesome and uplifting way. The scale showed an unexpected 231 pounds which meant I had lost 4 pounds in just one night! Although I know today that this is not possible and that the 4 pounds could have been a number of things such as water weight or undigested food, I did not know any of it then and chose to believe my workout from the previous night had magically yielded fast results. It was all the motivation I needed and the next thing I did was put on my running shoes and go back to the gym for another run. I weighed myself again later that day and weighed even less. And that is how my long journey to weight loss began.

But enough about me. This book is about you and your journey to fitness. What follows is a step by step guide to embarking on that journey and implementing an effective and sustainable weight loss routine. You are about to learn the day to day lifestyle adjustments that helped me and tens of other men and women lose extreme amounts of weight in a relatively short time. But do not thank me just yet. Just keep reading.

The 5 Step Guide to Fast and Simple Weight Loss:

Step 1: Assessing Yourself and Your Many Problems

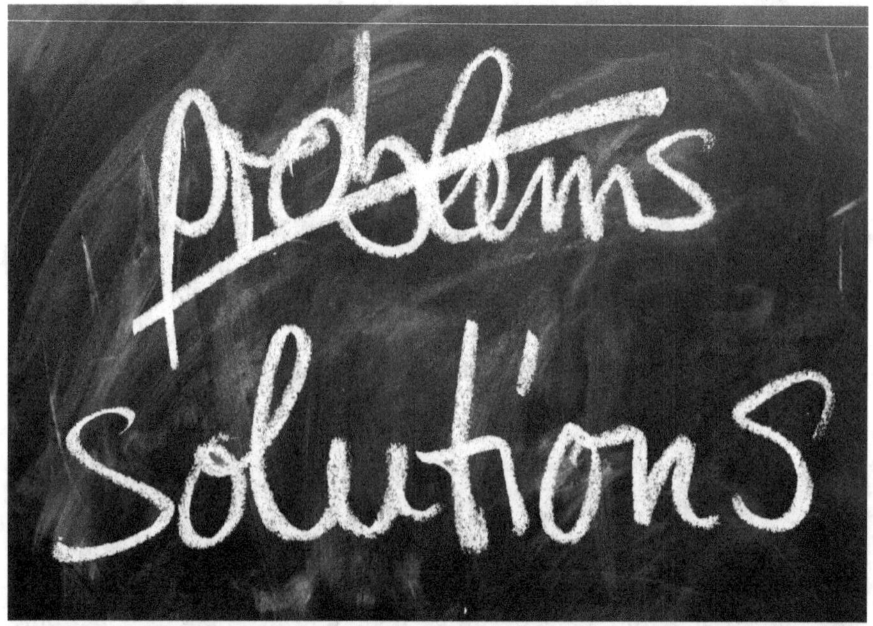

"If you know your enemies and know yourself, you will not be imperiled in a hundred battles." – Sun Tzu

Believe it or not, the main reason you are struggling with weight loss, the main reason you have weight to lose in the first place, is You. Yes, on your journey to weight loss, you are going to be your biggest enemy. And in order to vanquish the bad binging urges and the laziness to workout, you will need to asses who you are, right now, and who you want to become. And this is exactly what step 1 is for.

In this first step, we are going to go over a number of problems that have put you in the situation you are in, and are making it hard for you to get out of it. Before we start, make sure you have access to a mirror. You are going to need it to complete this first step. Now, let's go over these *problems*.

Problem #1: You are an addict

I am sure you are familiar with the feeling I mentioned a few paragraphs ago. The excitement you get at the prospect of gobbling an entire pint of chocolate chip cookie dough Ben&Jerry's ice cream. I am sure you are even more familiar with the feeling of disgust that comes towards the end of a bad meal. And what about the new resolutions you often come up with to make yourself feel better? I am sure you know exactly what I am talking about. Things like "Okay, from now on, no more carbs" or "Starting tomorrow, I am going to exercise every day and eat healthy". But for some reasons, these resolutions only last a few hours, until the next opportunity to eat junk presents itself. That is when you go back to rationalizing, convincing yourself that it is not that big of a deal and that you can make up for it later. It is a pattern that all addicts experience. Yes, if you did not know then this is the first bit of news I have for you. You are, whether you believe it or not, an addict. And you are not just addicted to food. Humans are, by nature, addicted to food, which is in no way a problem. It is actually a healthy addiction. The thing you are addicted to is poor nutrition. You are addicted to meals and quantities of food that are poisonous to your health. You are addicted to junk food. You are literally a junkie. If you do not believe me, take a second to answer the following question. Are you aware that eating junk food is bad for you? If not, then I have bad news for you. Eating junk food is bad for you. But I am quite sure you already knew that. So now ask yourself this. If you know that junk food is bad for you, why do you eat it so often? Why do you regularly consume foods that you know are detrimental to your health? Are you suicidal? Or is it simply too good and tasty for you to turn down? I am guessing the latter. And that is how you know that you are an addict. When you get so much pleasure out of doing something life threatening that you ignore the dangers associated with it. When you can't even think rationally and do what is best for you in moments of temptation. You probably know someone who keeps saying they are going to quit smoking. But for some reason, they always seem to be smoking their "last cigarette". Maybe that someone is you. In any case, you have to understand that this is the exact same problem you have with junk food. You are addicted. And this addiction makes it impossible for you to stop eating when you are full, or to start eating healthier foods. But what do addicts do when they realize they have a problem? They seek help, which is exactly what you are doing by reading this book. Congratulations! Now is the time to get better. And the first step of addiction recovery is *honesty*. So put this book down right now and complete the following exercise. Well, read the instructions first, then put the book down.

Exercise 1: Self-Assessment

Look around you and find a mirror. Any type of mirror works. You can even use your iPhone screen if it is the closest thing you have to a mirror. Once you have found a mirror, look yourself in it for a few seconds and say, out loud: "Hi, my name is (*your name*), and I am an addict." I am serious. Put down your kindle device right now, and go do what I just explained. You can come back in a few seconds.

Done? Good. Now that you have admitted one of your many problems, it is time to move over to your next big problem: boredom.

Problem #2: You are bored

There is a reason you spend so much of your time with food in your mouth. It is because you often have the opportunity to. You are often in a situation where eating seems like the only logical thing to do. You are often bored. Yes. It may seem overly simple but it is true. I could have easily listed this as problem number one. And here is the thing. Life, in itself, can be extremely boring. And that is okay. Part of being human is feeling bored at times. In fact, we can't always be doing something. We can't spend 24 hours at work. We can't always have friends to hang out with. We can't always come up with fun activities to engage in. And the problem with people like you and me is that when we run out of ideas for things to do, our first reflex is to look for something to put in our mouths. We mistake boredom for hunger because food has always given us temporary releases of pleasure. But there is a crucial difference between being hungry and wanting to eat. We are hungry when our body needs food to function. We want to eat when we are bored. And it takes serious willpower to fight the urge to eat when we feel like it. So it is important that you always remember the following equation:

Boredom – Willpower = Unnecessary Binging

What is willpower? What does it mean to be willing? To want something. Think about it. Do you really want to lose weight? To change?

Problem #3: You do not really want to lose weight, YET

I believe the answer is NO! Let me explain. There is a big difference between thinking you want something and actually wanting that thing. For instance, we would all love to be billionaires. We would all like to be loved and admired by everyone. We would all love to be fit and healthy all the time. But do we actually want any of those things. I do not believe so. In my opinion, if you will not do the things necessary to get something, then you do not really want it. Indeed, to want something does not mean to fantasize about it. It means to go after it. Will is not a thought, a wish, or a desire. Will is an action. And that is a very important thing to realize. The phrase "I want to, but I can't" is one of the most idiotic and nonsensical things you can ever say or think. It is a lame excuse. A way to rationalize and exist with yourself without regret and disappointment. I used to think I could never be thin. I used to think I could never get six pack abs. I used to think I could never get a girlfriend. Today, I have achieved all of the above. And the only difference between me now and me then is *Action*. I eat healthy, I workout regularly, and I approach people without fear. That is all that has changed. I did not drink any magic protein shake, and I wasn't bitten by any radioactive insect. I just decided I actually wanted things I did not have and took action to get them. So take a few seconds to answer the following questions: Do you really want to lose weight? Do you really want to forgo all the tasty dishes you are so used to savouring on a regular basis? Do you really want to sweat, be sore, and push yourself to the limit? Do you really want to get out of your comfort zone? Or, are you so comfortable now that you would actually rather settle for who you currently are? There is nothing wrong with that by the way. It is what you are doing now, so clearly, it is what you want now. Unfortunately, you can't have it both ways. You can't want to be comfortable and want to be an improved version of yourself at the same time. The following exercise will help put you in an action taking state of mind.

<u>Exercise 2: What do you want?</u>

Once again, I want you to put down this book and walk over to the mirror. Look yourself in it for a few seconds. Ask yourself. ***What do I want?*** Do I want to lose weight? Is it worth all the sacrifices? Is it worth all the pain? What am I getting out of it? What are my motivations. How will it make my life better? Complete this exercise and come back.

Done? Good! How do you feel after that one on one exchange with yourself? Did you realize that you do not actually want to lose weight? If so, that is fine. Just put down the book, for good this time, and go live your life. Stop obsessing about the idea of losing weight. Just live with the decision you made to be the way you currently are, and stop adding extra stress to your life. You really do not need it, and neither does your heart. I do not know you, but I am sure you are a great person, so you should learn to love yourself just the way you are.

If, on the other hand, you realized that it is time for a change and you actually decided that you ***Want*** to lose weight, Congratulations! You have made it to **Step 2**.

Step 2: Finding your True Motivation(s)

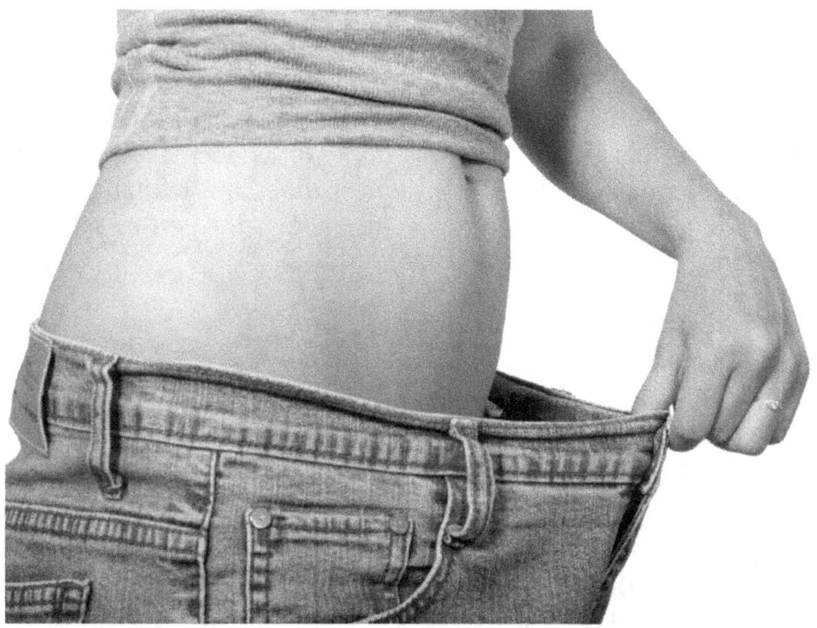

"People often say that motivation does not last. Well, neither does bathing - that is why we recommend it daily." – Zig Ziglar

For this step, you are going to need a place to sit or lie down, and relax. A bed would be perfect, but a couch or even a chair would work as well. You are probably already using one of these anyway so you should be good. If you think it is comfortable enough for you to relax, then you are all set. If not, go find something comfy enough and come back. Also, if you have an iPod or any mp3 player, you can use it. I personally find it helpful for completing this exercise. Got everything? Good!

The great thing about finding the right motivation is that it is an excellent drive. It also makes the weight loss effort more enjoyable. It enables you to dream, to visualize the future you want, and embrace it before it even happens. Without the right motivations, I probably would not have lost a single pound. Every tasteless meal I had, every mile I ran, it was all accompanied by this vision. This dream of my new body, the compliments, the constant validation from people around me. And it kept me going every day.

So ask yourself what it is you are really after. Why it is that you are willing to sacrifice so much just to get in shape. And one thing to keep in mind is that there is no such thing as a good or a bad motivation. There are just motivations. It can be as shallow as "I want to impress this girl" which was mine, or as deep as "I want to be the best version of myself possible". It does not matter. Find a motivation that is genuine and powerful enough for you to actually want to work for it.

<u>Exercise 3: Start Fantasizing</u>

All right. Now is the time to lie/sit down, and relax. Read the following instructions before you close your eyes and apply them. If it helps, take your iPod and play a tune that relaxes you, makes you feel good, and helps you dream easier. Find a relaxing position. Any position that you enjoy works. Then relax and let all of the tension in your body go away. Do not fall asleep though. Once you find a comfortable position, close your eyes and start picturing yourself in a few months. Picture your amazing body. Picture people's amazement at the sight of this new you. Picture all the confidence coming your way and embrace it. Take deep breaths. Be as specific as you can. Picture your number one motivation for losing weight. The girl/guy you are trying to get with, the people you are trying to impress, or just the state of mind you are trying to be in. Picture all the positivity that will come from you achieving this faraway goal. And just stay there, for 5 minutes or so, eyes closed. Let your imagination go wild. Let the crazy thoughts come to you. The more unrealistic the better. Just lose yourself in that fantasy and come back in a few minutes. Again, do not fall asleep.

Are you back? How was it? Awesome right? I really enjoy this exercise. I usually do it when I am walking, jogging, or on the train. I just listen to music, and dream of the future. Not only is it fun, it keeps me motivated to do the things I have to do to make all my fantasies come true. But anyway. Now that we are back to reality, here is what you need to realize. All those things you dreamed can and will come true. All of them, down to the very last detail. You just have to make them happen. I used the word "dream" because I know how impossible it seems to you. It seems unrealistic, far away, and you feel like no matter how strongly you believe it, you are never going to burn all that belly fat and get a flat stomach. Well, take it from me, it will happen! I guarantee it. There is a 100% chance that you will get the body you want. I usually would not be this optimistic, but the very fact that *I,* of all people, achieved something so difficult, is the proof that anybody can achieve weight loss.

From now on, all you have to do is remember this feeling you got from fantasizing and carry it with you in everything you do, everywhere you go. Repeat the exercise as many times as necessary for the dream to be imbedded in your everyday reality. Soon enough, it will come naturally to you and help you get through tough workouts and tofu meals.

Step 3: Understanding the Real Goal

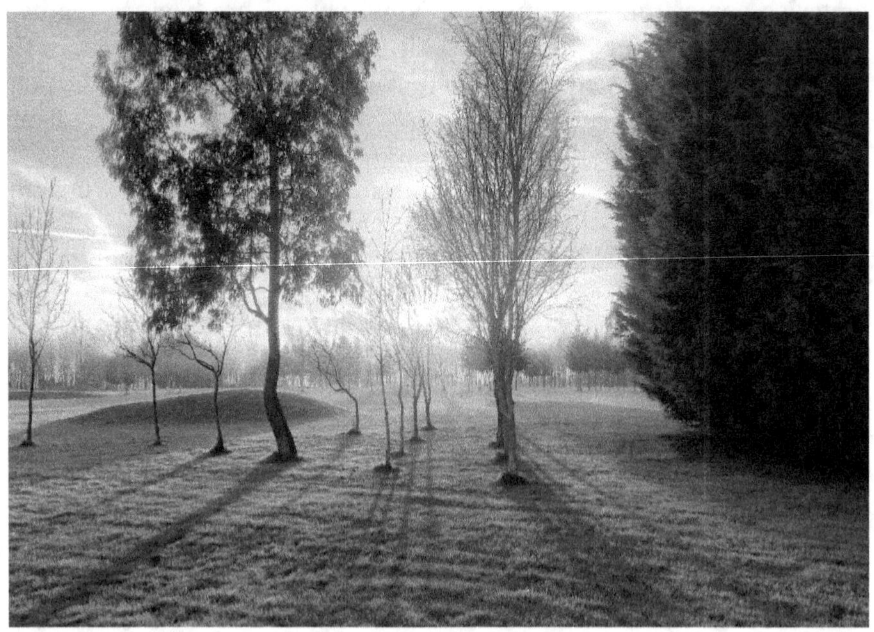

"Never give up. Today is hard, tomorrow will be worse, but the day after tomorrow will be sunshine." – Jack Ma

At this point, you have decided that you want to get in shape and you know the reason why. You now have a clear goal in mind which is a crucial part of you reaching it someday. But that day is not today, nor tomorrow, nor the day, the week, or the month after that. That day is just someday. You can't plan for it; you can't decide when it is going to be. But as long as you consistently apply the guidelines in this book, it will just happen, magically. You will wake up one day, look yourself in the mirror, and see the body you have been dreaming of for so long. So again, it is not a tangible goal nor is it a close one. The good news is, there is an even more important goal that is within your immediate reach. That goal is Today. Being able to follow a disciplined game plan today, without faltering, without cheating. That should be your main focus. Going to bed having accomplished everything you had set out to when you woke up. And the great thing about today, and tomorrow's today, and the today after that is that they add up. Yes, this dream of yours, this fantasy you have that seems so far away, this fit and lean body you want, this big ambitious goal is nothing but the sum of your todays. So take every day as its own destination, as its own accomplishment, as its own goal. And keep in mind that if you made it through today, you are one step closer to your goal. That as long as you get your todays right, reaching the perfect weight is only a matter of time. A promise. A guarantee. It is just like Confucius said "A journey of a thousand miles begins with a single step". So start your journey today and enjoy it, one step at time, with patience and confidence. When you get out of your house to go visit friend, you never worry about getting there. You know the way and you know that as long as you keep walking or driving, you will get to your destination eventually. The exact same applies to your journey to weight loss. There is nothing to doubt or worry about. As long as you take a new step every single day, you will get there.

Step 4: The 10 Lifestyle Adjustments for Fast and Simple Weight Loss

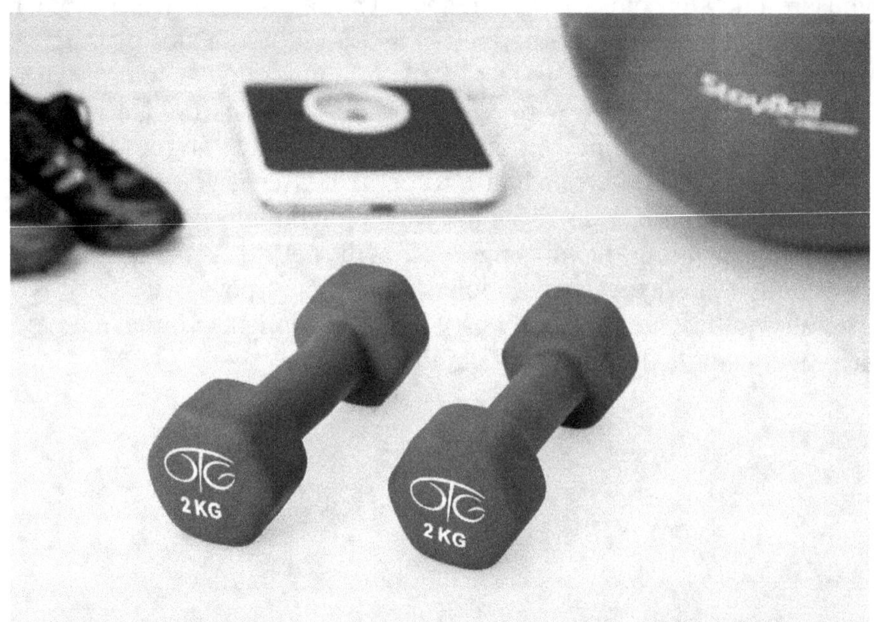

"The soul, like the body, accepts by practice whatever habit one wishes it to contact" – Socrates

Now that you understand the importance of patience and consistency, I am going to give you the actual adjustments you are going to make to your daily routine to lose weight effectively. In time, these adjustments will become habits that will enable you to naturally get fit and stay fit. I ask that you thoroughly read through the following guidelines, make sure you understand every single one of them, and start applying them today!

Adjustment #1: Find your proper calorie intake

You are probably familiar with the saying *"You are what you eat"*. This is absolutely 100% true. When it comes to getting in shape, nutrition accounts for about 80% of the work. In other words, if you want to get in shape, you have to eat well, and you have to eat right. It is hard, especially considering all the things you enjoy eating that you will not be eating for a while. But it is all worth it. What I want you to do is go on Google and lookup "calorie calculator". There are many different websites you can use and it does not really matter which one you pick. I would recommend using **http://caloriecontrol.org/healthy-weight-tool-kit/assessment-calculator/**. It is simple enough and serves the purpose you need it for. Open up the site and enter all the necessary data into the calculator provided (your weight, your height, your age, etc.). Under "Activity Level" select "Sedentary". You will see why in a bit. When you are done, submit the data you just entered, and collect the results. It should tell you how many calories you need to consume on a daily basis in order to maintain your current weight.

Now take that number, subtract **500** from it, and jot it down on a piece of paper. For example, I am **6'0** tall and used to weigh **235 pounds**. I needed around **2511 calories** a day to maintain my weight at the time, so I planned to consume **2011**instead. Again, record the number returned by the online calculator, subscribe 500 from it, and you are all set. This will guarantee that you burn at least 500 extra calories every day, which adds up to **3500 calories a week**, which evaluates to **a pound lost per week**. Yes, it is that simple.

Adjustment #2: Come up with a proper meal plan

Now that you know exactly how many calories you should be consuming every day, it is time to make sure you do not exceed that value. A simple way to do so is to ask the most knowledgeable person you know, Google. This time, lookup "**low calorie meal plans**" or "**low calorie meals**", and do the math to find a plan that does not exceed your daily calorie limit. This is a pretty good link for such recipes**http://www.eatingwell.com/nutrition_health/weight_loss_diet_plans/diet_meal_plans/7_day_diet_meal_plan_to_lose_weight_1200_calories** , but there are many more you can use. The choice is yours. Make sure to select meals that are easy enough for you to make, and varied enough that you do not get sick of them. Also, make sure you currently have or can easily get the necessary ingredients to cook them. Once that is done, make a spreadsheet, with 7 columns for days of the week, and 3 rows for meals of the day (breakfast, lunch, dinner), and populate that spreadsheet with your different meal choices. Again there are many software options available, but I would recommend using *Excel*. Once you have your meal plan in a clear table format, print it and stick it to your fridge, wall, or anywhere you have easy access to it.

Adjustment #3: Get rid of all the junk

This is one of the hardest things you will have to do in the next few months. I want you to go to your kitchen and search through all your stuff. Open your fridge along with all your cupboards, and take out everything that you know is junk. Cheetos, cookies, Nutella, pizza leftovers, frozen French fries, ice cream, bread, pretty much anything that is not a fruit or a vegetable. Just take it all out and put it on a table. Now look at it for a few seconds and remember the decision you made a few pages ago. "I want to lose weight. I want to change". Think about your fantasy. Remember how happy it makes you. Then find a trash bag, and dump all the junk in it. Once the table is all clear, take the trash bag you just filled and make sure to throw it somewhere outside of your house, either in a trash bin or in the garbage area of your building. Just make sure it is outside of your home. Like I said before, this is hard and extreme. But it must be done. Just do it and do not think about it too much. I realize you probably feel like you are throwing away tens of dollars but believe me, you can't put a price on fitness. What you can also do is give it away to a homeless person, a charity close to your home, or a neighbor. Anything you chose to do with that trash bag is fine as long as you no longer have access to it.

Adjustment #4: Do groceries

Now that you have cleared some useful space, it is time to fill up again. This is a very important adjustment. You have to get in the habit of doing groceries regularly in order to ensure you always have something to cook with. You have to do groceries at least once a month, without fail. Get all the ingredients you need to satisfy your meal plan requirements, and use them until you run out. Also, try never to do groceries on an empty stomach, you will tend to get more than you actually need due to hunger. Fruits are a crucial component of your grocery list. Get whichever ones you like the most, and make sure you have enough to eat a minimum of **3 fruits a day** (21 a week).

Adjustment #5: Change the way you eat and enjoy it

I know. I just made you throw away things you really enjoy eating. But believe me, that was the hardest part. And here is why. From now on, you are going to learn to enjoy everything you eat, no matter what it is or is not made of. It may not seem doable but it absolutely is. Take me for instance. I used to hate carrots, peas, and spinach. I would avoid all meals that included them. Today, I can't get enough of these vegetables. In fact, I eat carrots, peas, and spinach at least once a day. What changed? I learned to love them. It was very hard at first. Having to chew on things that seemed so blend and unappealing was quite a chore. And I used to think to myself "There is no way I can keep up with this. This is not food". But as time went by and I started familiarizing myself with different cooking variations of these ingredients, they began to grow on me. And the key to achieving this is to actually savor your food instead of just gobbling it. So from now on, you are going to savor every single meal you have. The following eating adjustments will help you eat healthier and enjoy it.

Eating Adjustment #1: Cook your own meals

This is crucial. Part of learning to enjoy your meals is to cook them yourself. It is hard to explain but there is a certain willingness to enjoy food when it resulted from your own work. It is rewarding. It will also help you develop the discipline to cook every single day without it feeling like a chore. Eventually, you will learn to enjoy the process. It will also reduce the incentive to eat takeout, which is as costly as it is unhealthy.

Eating Adjustment #2: Make reasonable portions

Again, refer back to your meal plan and calorie limit. Most recipes you will find online come with precise measurements for each ingredient you need to use. Do not exceed those measurements. Even if you feel like the portions you are making are too small, trust science and trust math. These portions are exactly what you need to survive, so do not make any more.

Eating Adjustment #3: Take your time and do not try to get full

My grandmother always used to say: "*eating is not a race*". And she was right. For your next meal, I want you to make sure you eat slowly and chew your food long enough. Develop the habit of taking smaller bites, and take the time to enjoy the contact of food with your tongue. It is scientifically proven that it takes about 20 minutes for your brain to get the information from your stomach that you are full. In other words, it is very easy for you to eat more than your body requires without knowing it. That is why you need to eat slowly. So that when your body has had enough, you get the information and stop.

Eating Adjustment #4: Always drink water. Stay away from sodas and juices

Sodas and juices are full of sugars and very toxic chemicals that make it hard for you to lose weight. The average man needs about 37.5 grams (9 teaspoons) of added sugar per day in order to function properly while women require about 25 grams (6 teaspoons). A regular can of coke contains about 40 grams of sugar. In other words, a single can of soda exceeds the amount of added sugar your body needs for a whole day. That is why drinking juices and sodas is incredibly dangerous. All they do is significantly increase your calorie intake and slow down your weight loss mechanism. So stay away from sugary beverages and get into a water only diet. Make sure you drink as much of it as you can, even when you are not thirsty. Water is a proven metabolism booster and great for maintaining your health. It also helps you feel more full when eating and thus, keeps you from going overboard with your meals. When consumed in moderation, coffee and tea can also be excellent substitutes for sodas and juices. Just do not add any sugar to them.

Eating Adjustment #5: Cut carbs like a crazy ex

This one was the hardest for me. I always used to have at least two slices of bread with everything I ate. I could not imagine my life without bread. The simple thought of having a meal without it was disgusting to me. But I had to do it. For the greater good. Cut your carb intake and keep your consumption of bread, rice, pasta, and cakes to a minimum. It is hard to get rid of them entirely. But again, the goal here is for you to learn to savor the foods you eat without all the unhealthy enhancers you are used to such as carbs and sugar. Replace them with healthy ones: peas, corn, Brussel sprouts, spinach, fruits, and other vegetables.

Eating Adjustment #6: Do not eat and watch TV/Movies at the same time

I really do not know why but for some reason, watching television shows, movies, or YouTube videos, while eating, has always made me binge-eat. It is like my brain associates the action of watching something entertaining with putting food in my mouth. So just to make sure the same thing does not happen to you, avoid all kinds of screens while you are eating. Focus on the food in front of you instead. Contemplate the result of your hard work. Watch the ingredients intertwined with one another. Appreciate the taste their combination creates in your mouth as you chew and swallow. This is all the entertainment you need.

And that is it. Apply these 6 eating adjustments and you will start to eat much better. And remember, nutrition is the most important aspect of fitness. The other one is exercise which we will get into next.

<u>Adjustment #6: Gear up</u>

Exercise does not necessarily mean extreme workouts. You do not have to push yourself beyond your limits. The goal behind exercising is to make sure you consistently burn more calories than you usually would in a day. So what you need to do now is go to the sports store closest to you and get running shoes, running shorts, and tops you feel comfortable running in. Get enough of each item to run 7 times a week. If you already have all that stuff, even better.

<u>**Adjustment #7: Run!**</u>

That is right. I said 7 time a week! You need to Run **Every Single Day**. Although I recommend running in the morning, you can pick any time of the day that works for you and stick to it. Every day. Do not make any excuses. Rain, shine, snow. No matter what. Always go for that run. You can gear up for any weather that is not extreme.

Again, the goal is not to engage in intense physically excruciating exercises. All I want you to do is allocate 15 to 20 minutes of each day to a running routine. Nothing too intense, just a light jog, preferably in the morning, when you wake up, before you eat anything. If necessary, set your alarm to 30 minutes earlier than usual so you have the time to workout without pressure. Also, remember always to stretch before you run. It is good for your muscular health.

Your workout routine should rely on two crucial and fundamental principles: *consistency* and *progress*. You will achieve the first one by making the decision, every morning, to get out of bed, gear up, and go for a run. That is it.

As far as progress, you will achieve it by running a little more everyday than you did the day before. How much more? It is all up to you. Just let it be more, and be honest with yourself. Chances are, you will not be able to run for too long at first. Again, this is nothing to worry about. You are out of shape which is the reason for you doing all this. Just keep in mind that the worst a shape you are in, the more room for improvement there is. And this is where the fun part begins. Let's say you go for a run tomorrow morning and find yourself out of breath after only 3 minutes. That is okay. 3 minutes is not much, but it is a start. And the way to progress from a 3-minute run is to run for 4 minutes the next day, and so on. When I started jogging, I could only run 6 minutes before feeling depleted. And it made me feel bad because I knew I wasn't running much. I could see other people running around the gym track for tens of minutes without showing any signs of fatigue. So what did I do? I motivated myself the way I showed you a few pages ago. I started fantasizing. I pictured myself months down the line, running at their pace, for even longer. And I slowly but incrementally started running more, and more, and more. By the end of the first two months, I could run for 20 minutes without stopping. Then 30, and so on. Today, I run 9 miles in 70 minutes every other day. I am in the best shape of my life, and the 6 minutes that used to get me so out of breath aren't even enough to get me warmed up. I have literally come a long way and so will you.

Again, be consistent, progress, and more importantly, **Run**! And remember, **No Excuses**. If you are sleepy, still get up and run. If you are unmotivated, fantasize, get up and run. If you feel hungry, definitely get up and run. Do not let anything be an excuse for you not to run every single day. Excuses are the enemy. If you make one today, chances are you will tomorrow. And the day you start making excuses is the day you ruin all your chances of consistency. I am not asking you to lift extreme weights or go rock climbing. I am just asking you to Run, which is much easier than it sounds.

Adjustment #8: Get new hobbies

Of all the adjustments you have to make, this is by far the easiest one. There are so many different activities you can engage in that will capture your interest and keep you from feeling bored. Remember, boredom is a major problem, and you can't let it happen because that is when you will turn to unnecessary binging. And again, finding new hobbies is easy. I picked up a few on my journey to fitness such as meditation, chess, Improv, and blogging. If any of these sound remotely interesting to you, I would recommend giving them a try. I am sure you will enjoy them more than you think. If not, then explore other possibilities. Again, your options are infinite. Once you find one or many activities you enjoy, try to do them as regularly as possible. Never let boredom get to you in between meals. Never. And if you just can't seem to find anything interesting enough, then go for a walk, or even an extra run every now and then. Why not?

Adjustment #9: Get a scale

If there is one thing more motivating than a fantasy, it is actual results. In order to stay motivated and constantly remind yourself that you are on the right track, get in the habit of weighing yourself once a week. No more. There are so many factors impacting your weight fluctuation such as water retention, sleep duration, or time of the day that weighing yourself every single day does not make sense. You would never get an accurate idea of how much you actually weigh and how much weight you have actually lost unless you give your body enough time to process its own changes.

Adjustment #10: Change the Rules of the game

At this point, you are probably overwhelmed by all the information I have shared with you. If so, do not worry, it is quite normal. The remainder of this book will somewhat summarize everything you have learned so far, and help you structure your day to day journey to fitness. One very helpful way to remember all these adjustments is to establish clear rules and thoroughly follow them. This will train your brain to automatically condemn destructive behavior while encouraging beneficial actions. I recommend typing them down or writing them on a piece of paper. It can be helpful to refer to these rules every day. Although I numbered them, there is no real order of importance as each one of these rules is crucial for you to attain your weight loss goals.

Rule #1: Run!
Rule #2: Never make excuses.
Rule #3: Always take the stairs. Avoid elevators and escalators.
Rule #4: For short distances, always take the walking option instead of the bus.
Rule #5: Cook your own meals every single day.
Rule #6: Drink water all the time. Even when you are not thirsty.
Rule #7: Stick to your meal plan and respect quantities.
Rule #8: Limit yourself to your meal plan. Do not eat anything outside of it except for fruits.
Rule #9: Snack on fruits every single day.
Rule #10: Savor your food. Do not gobble. Take the time to enjoy your meals.
Rule #11: Always do something in between meals. Never let yourself get bored.
Rule #12: No more cookies, chips, and unhealthy mass produced snacks.
Rule #13: No more sodas and juices. Remember **Rule #6**.

Rule #14: No unhealthy carbohydrates. Cut your consumption of bread, pasta, cakes, and rice.

Rule #15: Drink tea during and in between meals. You can also drink coffee in moderation.

Rule #16: Do not add sugar to anything you eat or drink.

Rule #17: No late night snacks. Make sure not to eat anything within 2 hours of your bed time.

Rule #18: Sleep. Make sure you get your 6 to 8 hours every day.

Rule #19: Do groceries at least once a month.

Rule #20: Never do groceries on an empty stomach.

Rule #21: Do not eat and watch TV/Movies/YouTube at the same time.

Rule #22: Weight yourself once a week. No more, no less.

Rule #23: If you cheat, do not get discouraged. But do not cheat again.

Some of these rules may seem extreme. Others useless. But you have to remember, it is the sum of the little things you do that makes for big changes. All the rules listed above worked for me and the many people I have coached over the years. I guarantee they will work for you.

Optional Adjustment: Get a Fitness Buddy

As you can probably tell by now, I give a lot of importance to motivation. I have already given you two tips to keep yourself motivated all throughout your journey to weight loss: fantasizing and tracking your progress. However, there is a third way to keep your drive alive and constantly fuel your efforts both mentally and physically: Finding a Fitness Buddy.

This is not a mandatory adjustment, and it is very possible to achieve weight loss without it. I did not have a fitness buddy when I lost weight. However, having one is an extremely helpful way to keep you going, and to prevent you from making excuses. From years of experience as a fitness coach, I have noticed that people who join my program in pairs are usually more motivated and consequently, achieve faster results. I have had the chance to coach couples, siblings, pairs of friends, and in most cases, their progress exceeds my initial expectations. And there is a clear reason for that. It is much easier to falter, make excuses, and give in to difficulties when the only person involved is you. You have no one to report to, and cheating only affects you, so it is not that big of a deal. However, having someone to share your endeavor with on a day to day basis reduces the incentive to cheat. You can't take a step back because they are moving forward, and they can't take a step back because you are moving forward. It creates a healthy spirit of competition that helps you lift each other up. It also helps to have someone who can immediately empathize when going through a tough workout, or when feeling muscle soreness. You are doing something hard but you are doing it together, which makes the stakes much higher, and the task much easier to tackle. It is no longer about you or them, it is about achieving a goal together.

So take a second to ask yourself: Who do I know that would be willing to do this with me? It can be anybody. They do not necessarily have to be overweight or looking to lose weight. They just have to have a pair of hands for cooking, and legs for running. Just ask anybody you think you could have a good time doing this with. A close friend, a spouse, a boyfriend/girlfriend, one of your children, or even someone you do not know that well who might be interested. Just approach them with the idea and let them know what it is you are trying to accomplish. Share your plan for weight loss with them or just lend them this book.

What's in it for them? Fitness! Yes, no matter how good a shape they are in, that person can always benefit from regular workouts and healthy meals. Fitness is not a destination, it is a journey, a lifestyle. It is one thing to get fit, it is a whole other thing to stay fit. So just ask someone, anyone you feel comfortable interacting with on a daily basis, and invite them to join you on your journey to fitness. Remember, anyone can be your fitness buddy.

Step 5: The "Today" Blueprint

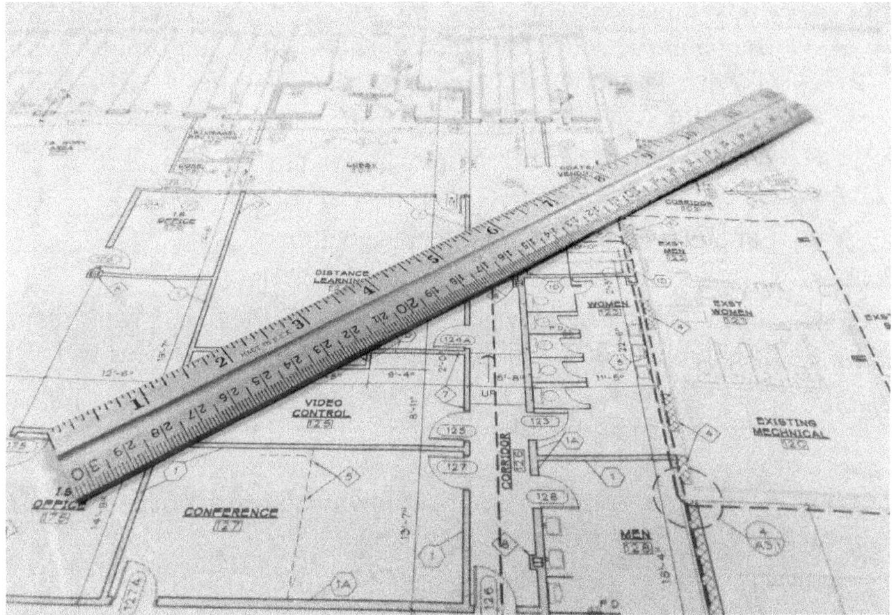

"The best preparation for good work tomorrow is to do good work today." – Elbert Hubbard

All right. Now that I have shared with you all my guidelines for weight loss, I want to go over everything one more time. I have developed the following blueprint to help you organize your days in a way that applies all the necessary adjustments. Make this your routine, stick to it and results are guaranteed to follow. Remember, every day is its own destination. Get your todays right and great tomorrows will magically follow.

The Today Blueprint:

- Wakeup earlier, early enough that you can go for a jog.
- Go for a jog and make sure you run more than you did the day before.
- Go over your meal plan for the day.
- Make breakfast.

- Eat breakfast.
- Start your day (Shower, work/school, etc.) and do not eat again until lunchtime (if somebody offers you donuts or cookies, politely decline and have tea or coffee instead).
- Cook Lunch (if you are going to spend your day outside of your home, cook your lunch ahead of time and bring it with you in a Tupperware). Again, respect quantities.
- Any time you feel hungry, eat fruits and drink water.
- Whenever you have free time, hobby up!
- At the end of your day, go home and cook dinner.
- Eat dinner at least 2 hours before bedtime.
- If any, keep leftovers for lunch the next day.
- If you have a buddy, get in touch with them and walk them through your day, step by step. Listen to their story as well.
- Go to sleep.
- Wake up and do it all again.

Again, it might be helpful to jot this down and refer to it at the start of each day.

Conclusion: Taking your First Step

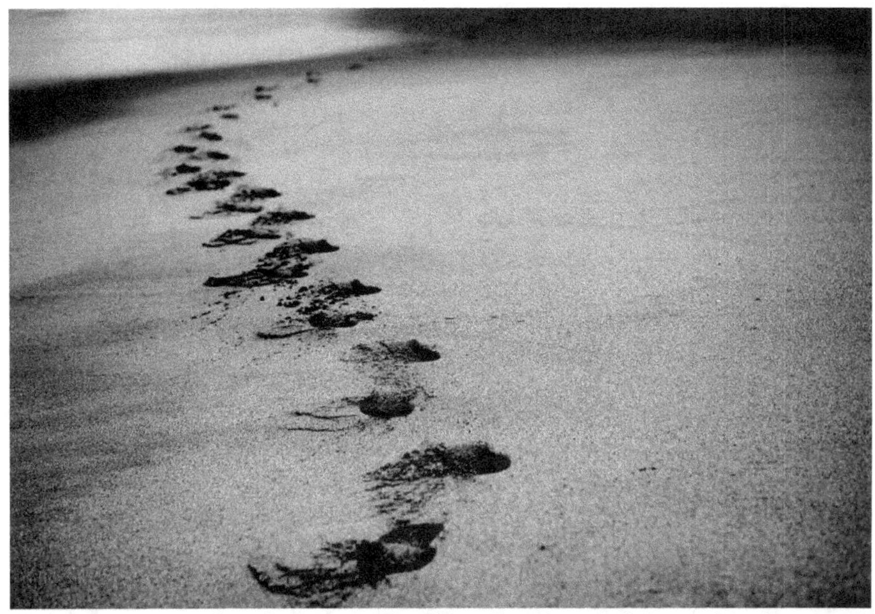

"A journey of a thousand miles begins with a single step"
– Confucius

At this point, I have shared with you everything I know about losing weight. I hope you found it helpful. The next and last thing I am going to ask you to do is to go back to the previous step "Today's Blueprint" and write every step of your day on a piece of paper. Once you are done, I want you to post pin it on your wall or use magnets to stick it to your fridge. Just anywhere you can easily access it every day. Then, I want you to find the guideline that is closest to the current time of your day and apply it right away. If you just woke up, put on your running shoes and go for a morning jog. **NOW!** If you are about to eat dinner, then do your low calorie planning now, and come up with a healthy and appropriate meal to eat before going to bed. Do not forget to wait at least two hours. Also, try to weigh yourself at some point during the day just so you can track your progress in the weeks to come. The most important part is to start now. Not tomorrow, not in a week, **RIGHT NOW!** If you do not start right away, you never will. Believe me. However, if you do start now, you will lose weight and be fit in no time. All you need is a decision. The rest will follow. Like magic. Taking that first step will drive the next one and so on. Soon, you will be going back to your mirror to contemplate and admire the beautiful body you have sculpted. Trust me.